ISBN: 978-965-7736-03-6

Disclaimer:

The information presented in this book represents the views of the publisher as of the date of publication. The publisher reserves the rights to alter update their opinions based on new conditions. This report is for informational purposes only. The author and the publisher do not accept any responsibilities for any liabilities resulting from the use of this information. While every attempt has been made to verify the information provided here, the author and the publisher cannot assume any responsibility for errors, inaccuracies or omissions. Any similarities with people or facts are unintentional.

Contents

Introduction

It's impossible to separate the history of the Turkish cuisine from the history of Turkey itself and its people. It is a well-known fact that the Turkish do not give up on their traditional foods easily, and for that reason we get to enjoy all these amazing foods. The Turkish people have taken care of their heritage and have passed the recipes from generation to generation, so that they survive in time, regardless of what those times bring. In addition, Turks are fairly conservative with their foods, and they follow strict customs and habits when it comes to their food.

But it shouldn't surprise us that Turkish cuisine is one of the greatest in the world. After all, Turkey is positioned in the Mediterranean area, and it has fertile grounds which allow people to grow vegetables and herbs. Turkey also has always been positioned in an area where it could easily gain control of most of the trade routes, so it had easy access to spices, herbs and ingredients that weren't available elsewhere. Such advantages helped develop a long lasting and influential cuisine.

There is a belief in Turkey that food is a symbol, and it often has established the social order. Turks were extremely protective with their territory in the past, but there were moments when they got together regardless of beliefs. Those moments were banquets and feasts where large amounts of foods were prepared, and everyone had a well-established role in order to make this happen. Large families often held feasts as a way of saying not only that they were rich, but also of stating that they are friendly and welcoming to people into their home. Giving food to your guests was a sign of good people, and those who shared their food with their guests were praised as important members of the society.

A few base ingredients seem to keep showing up in Turkish recipes, and one of these ingredients is wheat although sometimes it is replaced with barley, rice or millet. Wheat has been part of this cuisine for centuries, and it still represents one of the most consumed food in Turkey, either in the form of bread, flat bread, pilaf or desserts.

Vegetables were also a great part of the Turkish cuisine, although some of them were introduced in Turkey quite late, such as the eggplant. Turks adopted the eggplant and made it shine through dishes like Imam Baialdi. Apart from the eggplant the Turkish cuisine is similar to Mediterranean cuisine that relies heavily on fresh vegetables and plenty of herbs: tomatoes, bell peppers, zucchinis, olives, parsley and cilantro.

Dried fruits and nuts are also specific to Turkish cuisines. Originally introduced by the Persians, the Turks taught them how to cook wheat in return. By 1200 B.C. the Turkish Empire moved westward into Anatolia, where they encountered chickpeas, figs, olive oil and an abundance of seafood. We can say that the Turkish cuisine fully developed its characteristics in the mid 1400's when Turkish staples were developed: stuffed vegetables and salad, wrapped vegetables and rolls, thin sheets of dough and the use of spices in desserts.

APPETIZERS

Spiced Glazed Pecans

Spiced glazed pecans are what Turkish call meze and is served as an appetizer. They are spicy and ideal for a meal because they boost your digestion.

Time: 35 minutes
Servings: 6-8

Ingredients:

1 pound pecan halves
2 tablespoons water
1 tablespoon ground flax seeds
1 teaspoon salt
2 tablespoons agave syrup
1 teaspoon cinnamon powder
½ teaspoon ground cardamom
½ teaspoon ground star anise
½ teaspoon chili powder

Directions:

1. Mix the flax seeds, water, agave syrup and spices in a bowl.
2. Add the pecan halves and toss them around until well coated.
3. Spread the pecans on a baking sheet lined with parchment paper and cook in the preheated oven at 400°F for 20 minutes.
4. Serve the glazed pecans chilled.

Tofu Stuffed Jalapeños

Although traditionally made with cheese, these tofu stuffed jalapeños or green peppers still taste amazing. The spicy aroma infuses the tofu, and they complement each other perfectly.

Time: 40 minutes
Servings: 8

Ingredients:

   8 jalapeños or green peppers
   8 oz. creamy tofu
   1 tablespoon chopped chives
   ¼ teaspoon cumin powder
   2 garlic cloves, minced

Directions:

1. Cut the top of each pepper and carefully remove the seeds.
2. Mix the tofu, chives, cumin powder and garlic in a food processor and pulse until smooth.
3. Spoon the filling into each pepper. Secure the opening with a toothpick if needed.
4. Heat a grill pan over medium to high flame and place the peppers on the grill.
5. Cook the peppers on both sides until browned and serve them preferably warm.

Tofu Stuffed Jalapeños

Nothing compares to a spicy, fragrant stuffed jalapeño when it comes to waking up your taste buds!

Time: 40 minutes
Servings: 6

Ingredients:

   12 jalapeños
   8 oz. silken tofu
   2 green onions, chopped
   1 garlic clove, minced
   1 teaspoon turmeric powder
   Salt and pepper for taste
   1 tablespoon chopped parsley

Directions:

1. Pour the silken tofu in a bowl. Stir in the green onions, garlic, turmeric, parsley, salt and pepper.
2. Cut the top of each pepper and carefully remove the seeds.
3. Stuff each jalapeño with the tofu mixture and place them on a baking tray lined with parchment paper.
4. Cook in the preheated oven at 350°F for 20 minutes.
5. Serve the jalapenos warm or chilled.

Mediterranean Olives

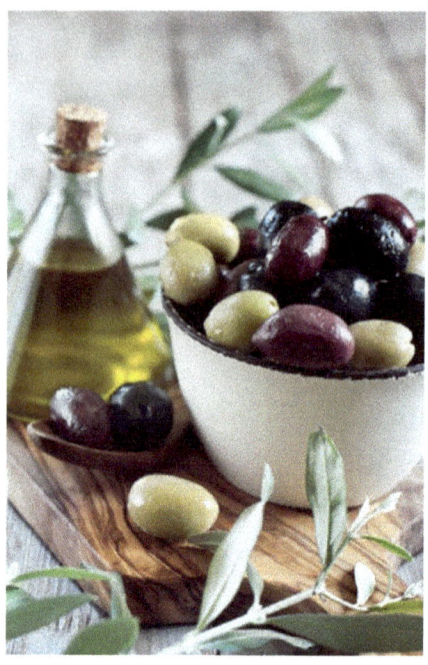

With this recipe you can make your own marinated olives at home. And you can customize the recipe any way you like!

Time: 15 minutes
Servings: 6-8

Ingredients:

    1 pound uncured black, green and Kalamata olives
    ½ cup sea salt
    ½ cup olive oil

Directions:

1. Combine all the ingredients in a glass jar.
2. Shake the jar well to evenly distribute the oil and salt.
3. Place the jar in a dark place for 25 days, shaking it once a day.
4. Serve the black olives after 25 days of marinating and curing.

Patates Mucveri – Potato Fritters

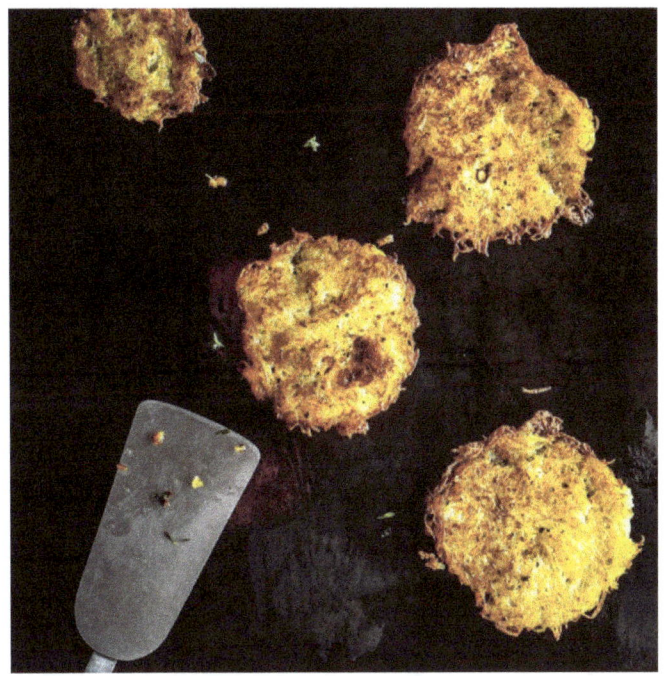

You got to love these filling, juicy potato fritters! Add fresh herbs for a flavor boost and a touch of red pepper for a heat kick.

Time: 40 minutes
Servings: 4-6

Ingredients:

1 pound red potatoes, peeled and grated
1 shallot, finely chopped
1 tablespoon chopped parsley
1 tablespoon chopped cilantro
2 tablespoons ground flax seeds
2 tablespoons cold water
Salt and pepper for taste
¼ teaspoon red pepper flakes
¼ cup vegetable oil for frying

Directions:

1. Combine all the ingredients in a bowl and mix well.
2. Heat the oil in a frying pan.
3. Drop spoonfuls of potato mixture into the hot oil and fry on each side for 3-4 minutes.
4. Place the fritters on paper towels and serve them warm or chilled.

Tofu and Red Pepper Spread

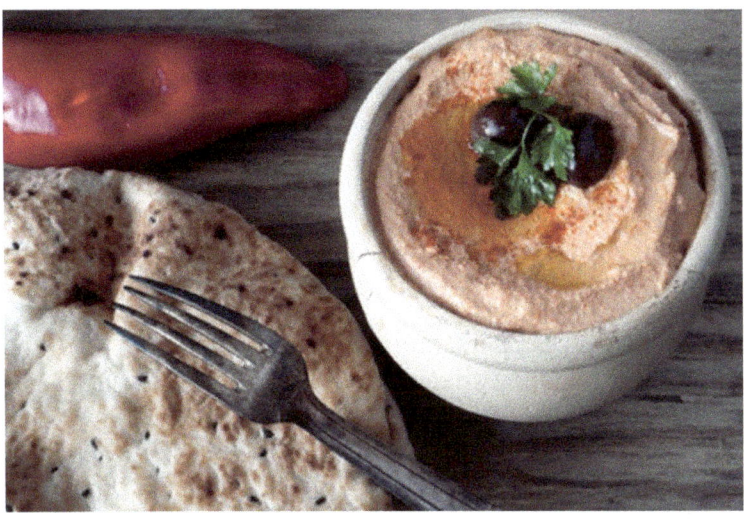

Although traditionally made with feta cheese, this recipe is just as good as the non-vegan version. It's slightly salty, but rich and delicious and amazing when served with crackers!

Time: 20 minutes
Servings: 4-6

Ingredients:

   4 roasted red bell peppers, drained
   8 oz. silken tofu
   2 garlic cloves
   1 tablespoon chopped shallot
   Salt and pepper for taste

Directions:

1. Combine all the ingredients in a blender and pulse until smooth.
2. Spoon the spread in a glass jar and store it in the fridge for 15 minutes.

Tofu Roasted Red Peppers

Mixing these roasted red peppers with tofu makes for a great dipping snack or appetizer.

Time: 30 minutes
Servings: 4-6

Ingredients:

4 oz. silken tofu
6 roasted red bell peppers, drained and chopped
2 tablespoons chopped cilantro
Salt and pepper for taste

Directions:

1. Mix the tofu with almond milk in a blender and pulse until smooth.
2. Pour the mixture into a bowl and stir in the bell peppers, cilantro, salt and pepper for taste.
3. Serve the appetizer fresh.

Sarimsakli Kuskonmaz - Garlicky Asparagus

You'll never see such an recipe again! For a dish to be ready in just a few easy steps, this one is incredibly delicious!

Time: 25 minutes
Servings: 4

Ingredients:

1 pound fresh asparagus, trimmed
3 tablespoons olive oil
2 garlic cloves, sliced
Salt and pepper for taste
2 tablespoons lemon juice

Directions:

1. Heat the oil in a skillet and stir in the garlic. Sauté for 30 seconds then remove the garlic.
2. Add the asparagus and cook on low heat for 15 minutes.
3. Season with salt and pepper then drizzle with lemon juice and serve the asparagus warm.

Cig Kofte

This raw appetizer is not something unusual for the Turkish cuisine. A bite of this and you get to know the essence of the Turkish food – tangy, garlicky and loaded with spices.

Time: 40 minutes
Servings: 4-6

Ingredients:

2 shallots, chopped
½ lemon, juiced
2 tomatoes, cubed
2 garlic cloves, chopped
2 tablespoons olive oil
½ teaspoon cumin seeds
½ teaspoon fennel seeds
1 cup bulgur, rinsed
3 cups hot water
2 tablespoons tomato paste
Salt and pepper for taste

Directions:

1. Mix the bulgur with water, tomato paste, salt and pepper in a saucepan and cook over medium flame for 15 minutes.
2. Remove from heat and let the bulgur soak up the liquid completely.
3. Stir in the remaining ingredients and adjust the taste with salt and pepper.
4. Serve the dish fresh.

Zucchini Potato Fritters

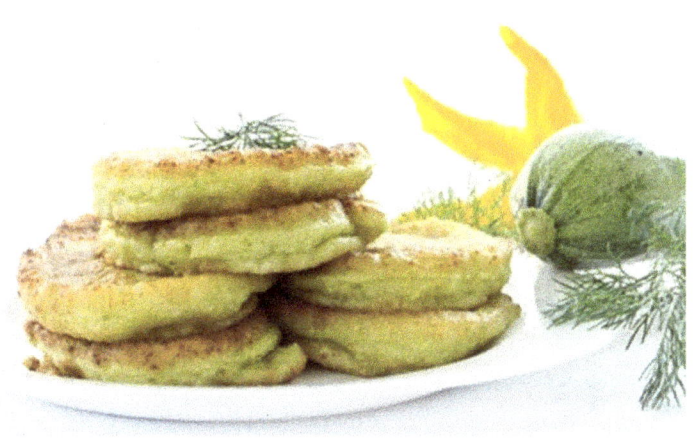

These mild fritters make an excellent appetizer for a family meal because they cover every single taste. Even the pickiest eaters will enjoy them!

Time: 40 minutes
Servings: 4-6

Ingredients:

3 red potatoes, peeled and grated
1 young zucchini, grated
1 tablespoon ground flax seeds
1 tablespoon water
¼ teaspoon cumin powder
¼ teaspoon red pepper flakes
1 shallot, chopped
Salt and pepper for taste
¼ cup vegetable oil for frying

Directions:

1. Mix the potatoes, zucchini, flaxseeds, water, cumin powder, red pepper flakes, shallot, salt and pepper in a bowl.

2. Heat the oil in a deep frying pan then drop spoonfuls of fritter mixture into the hot oil.
3. Fry them on both sides until golden brown.
4. Remove the fritters on paper towels and serve them warm or chilled.

Baba Ganoush

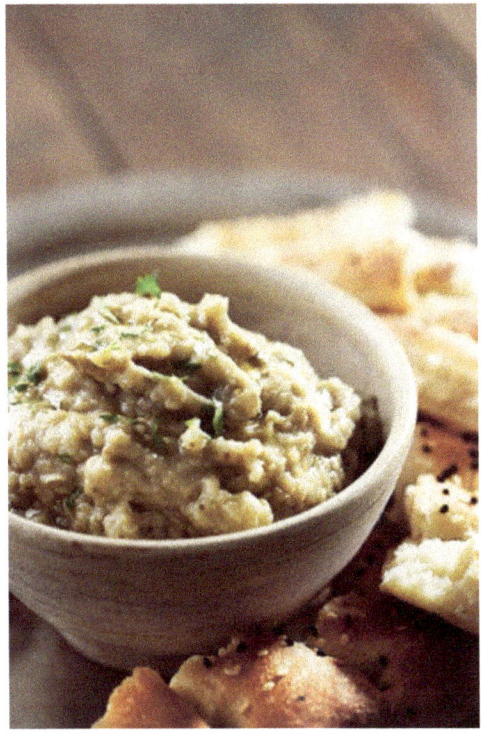

Without a doubt you've heard of baba ganoush before. It's a dip made with roasted eggplant, garlic and a touch of spices, and it's nothing but delicious!

Time: 1 hour
Servings: 2-4

Ingredients:

   1 large eggplant cut in half
   2 garlic cloves
   ½ shallot
   3 tablespoons olive oil
   Salt and pepper for taste
   1 tablespoon lemon juice

Directions:

1. Place the eggplant on a baking tray lined with parchment paper.
2. Cook in the preheated oven at 350°F for 35 minutes.
3. Spoon the soft flesh into a blender and add the garlic, shallot, olive oil, lemon juice, salt and pepper.
4. Pulse until smooth and serve the baba ganoush fresh.

Sautéed Spinach with Cashew Cream

The cashew cream brings the sautéed spinach to a whole new level, making it richer and more delicious!

Time: 30 minutes
Servings: 4-6

Ingredients:

　1 pound spinach, shredded
　3 tablespoons olive oil
　2 garlic cloves, minced
　1 shallot, chopped
　1 cup cashew nuts, soaked overnight
　2 tablespoons lemon juice
　¼ cup water
　Salt and pepper for taste

Directions:

1. Heat the olive oil in a skillet.
2. Add the garlic and shallot and sauté for 2 minutes.
3. Stir in the spinach and sauté for 15 minutes, stirring often.
4. While the spinach cooks, mix the cashew nuts, lemon juice and water in a blender and pulse until smooth.
5. Pour the mixture over the spinach then adjust the taste with salt and pepper.
6. Cook 5 additional minutes and serve the dish warm.

Caramelized Onions

Caramelized onions make an excellent appetizer in the Turkish cuisine, and you should give it a try before judging! You'll be surprised to discover a sweet, delicious appetizer!

Time: 30 minutes
Servings: 2-4

Ingredients:

5 red onions, sliced
¼ cup olive oil
½ teaspoon dried thyme
Salt and pepper for taste

Directions:

1. Heat the olive oil in a skillet.
2. Stir in the sliced onions and cook over medium flame for 20 minutes, stirring often, until the onions begin to caramelize.
3. Season with dried thyme, salt and pepper and serve the onions warm or chilled.

Garlicky Croutons

These croutons are an excellent treat on a buffet. They are loaded with garlic, olive oil and herbs and can be served alone or combined with other appetizers.

Time: 30 minutes
Servings: 4-6

Ingredients:

10 slices bread, cubed
¼ cup extra virgin olive oil
1½ teaspoons garlic powder
1 teaspoon dried Mediterranean herbs

Directions:

1. Spread the bread cubes in a baking tray lined with parchment paper.
2. Drizzle with olive oil then sprinkle with garlic powder and herbs.
3. Mix to evenly coat them and cook in the preheated oven at 400°F for 10-15 minutes, stirring once during the cooking process.
4. Let them cool in the oven for an even crispier texture.

Spiced Pecans

Time: 30 minutes
Servings: 4-6

Ingredients:

3 cups pecan halves
4 tablespoons coconut oil
½ teaspoon cinnamon powder
1 teaspoon cayenne pepper
½ teaspoon ground black pepper
1 teaspoon salt
¼ teaspoon ground ginger

Directions:

1. Spread the pecans in a baking tray lined with parchment paper.
2. Drizzle coconut oil over the pecans then sprinkle with cinnamon, cayenne pepper, black pepper, salt and ginger.
3. Cook in the preheated oven at 375°F for 15-20 minutes until fragrant and golden brown.
4. Let them cool in the pan before serving.

Muhammara – Turkish Red Dip

Muhammara is a traditional dip made with red peppers, walnuts, olive oil and pomegranate molasses which adds tanginess and color.

Time: 15 minutes
Servings: 4-6

Ingredients:

2 cups roasted red bell peppers
¼ cup breadcrumbs
¼ cup walnuts
2 garlic cloves
1 tablespoon pomegranate molasses
¼ cup olive oil
Salt and pepper for taste
Seed crackers for serving

Directions:

1. Combine all the ingredients in a blender or food processor.
2. Pulse until smooth then spoon the dip into a serving bowl.
3. Serve the dip with seed crackers.

Roasted Eggplant Dip with Cashews

Time: 45 minutes
Servings: 4-6

Ingredients:

1 eggplant
1 cup cashew nuts, soaked overnight
2 garlic cloves
¼ cup olive oil
Salt and pepper for taste

Directions:

1. Roast the eggplant in a preheated oven at 400ºF for 30 minutes until the skin is crisp and slightly burnt.
2. Remove from the oven and let it cool slightly then peel off the skin.
3. Place the flesh of the eggplant in a food processor.
4. Add the cashews, garlic, olive oil, salt and pepper and pulse a few minutes until smooth.
5. Pour the dip into a serving bowl and serve it fresh with crackers or bread.

Potato Tofu Salad

Although this recipe is simple, the outcome is delicious! Sometimes, simplicity is the best choice for a healthy and nutritious meal.

Time: 40 minutes
Servings: 4-6

Ingredients:

4 red potatoes, washed
6 oz. firm tofu, cubed
¼ cup olive oil
2 garlic cloves, minced
½ lemon, juiced
¼ cup chopped parsley
Salt and pepper for taste

Directions:

1. Boil the potatoes in a large pot of water until soft.
2. Peel the potatoes and cut them into cubes. Place them in a salad bowl.
3. Add the rest of the ingredients and stir gently.
4. Serve the salad as fresh as possible.

Sautéed Asparagus with Walnut Dressing

Turkish cuisine uses walnuts quite a lot, and this dish makes no exception. But it's the walnuts that make the dressing of this dish as rich and flavorful as it is.

Time: 40 minutes
Servings: 4-6

Ingredients:

1 pound fresh asparagus, trimmed
3 tablespoons olive oil
¼ cup walnuts
2 tablespoons lemon juice
2 tablespoons Dijon mustard
¼ teaspoon cumin powder
Salt and pepper for taste

Directions:

1. Heat the olive oil in a large skillet.
2. Place the asparagus in the hot oil and cook it for 15 minutes, stirring often.
3. To make the dressing, combine the walnuts, lemon juice, mustard and cumin powder in a small blender and pulse until smooth.
4. Pour the dressing over the asparagus and mix to evenly coat it.
5. Serve the asparagus warm or chilled.

Vegetable Stuffed Mushrooms

Mushrooms are a great meat replacer, and thankfully they are incredibly versatile. Choose medium size or small mushrooms to make sure your appetizers are bite-size!

Time: 45 minutes
Servings: 12

Ingredients:

12 small or medium size mushrooms
2 carrots, grated
1 shallot, chopped
2 tablespoons olive oil
½ teaspoon dried oregano
Salt and pepper for taste
½ cup cashew nuts, soaked overnight
1 tablespoon lemon juice

Directions:

1. Heat the oil in a skillet and stir in the carrots and shallot. Sauté for 5 minutes.
2. Remove the lower part of the mushrooms, wash them well and chop them. Then stir them into the hot oil.
3. Cook for 5 additional minutes then remove from heat and season with oregano, salt and pepper.
4. Mix the cashew nuts and lemon juice in a blender and pulse until smooth.
5. Spoon the filling into the mushroom caps and top with a dollop of cashew cream.
6. Cook in the preheated oven at 350°F for 30 minutes.
7. Let them cool in the pan before serving.

Roasted Bell Peppers in Tomato Sauce

If you use store bought roasted bell peppers for this dish, you cut down the cooking time a lot. But you get the same great and rich taste as with freshly roasted peppers.

Time: 30 minutes
Servings: 4-6

Ingredients:

2 tablespoons olive oil
1 shallot, chopped
2 garlic cloves, minced
2 cups tomato sauce
1 bay leaf
¼ teaspoon chili flakes
6 roasted bell peppers, halved
Salt and pepper for taste

Directions:

1. Heat the olive oil in a skillet.
2. Stir in the shallot and garlic and sauté for 2 minutes.
3. Add the tomato sauce, chili flakes and bell peppers, then season with salt and pepper.
4. Cook over low to medium flame for 20 minutes.
5. Let the dish cool completely before serving.

Stuffed Baked Potatoes

Don't neglect this recipe for being this simple! Sometimes simplicity it's what makes dishes taste amazing, and it's the simple combinations that yield great results.

Time: 55 minutes
Servings: 4

Ingredients:

   4 large red potatoes, washed
   1 teaspoon sweet paprika
   Salt and pepper for taste
   2 mushrooms, chopped
   1 garlic clove, minced
   ½ cup cashew nuts, soaked overnight
   2 tablespoons lemon juice
   2 tablespoons olive oil

Directions:

1. Season the red potatoes with salt, pepper and paprika and wrap each potato in aluminum foil.
2. Cook the potatoes in the preheated oven at 350°F for 40 minutes.
3. Mix the cashews with lemon juice and olive oil
4. Mix the mushrooms with garlic. Remove the potatoes from the oven and carefully un-wrap them.
5. Pierce the potatoes with a fork to make room for a dollop of mushrooms and cashew cream.
6. Place the potatoes back in the oven for an additional 10 minutes.
7. Serve the potatoes warm.

Shakshuka – Tofu in Tomato Sauce

Time: 40 minutes
Servings: 6

Ingredients:

   2 tablespoons olive oil
   1 shallot, sliced
   2 red bell peppers, cored and sliced
   1 can diced tomatoes
   1 cup tomato sauce
   1 bay leaf
   1 teaspoon Italian seasoning
   6 slices firm tofu
   Chopped cilantro for serving

Directions:

1. Heat the oil in a skillet and stir in the shallot. Sauté for 2 minutes.
2. Add the bell peppers, tomatoes, tomato sauce, bay leaf and seasoning and cook the sauce for 10 minutes.
3. Place the tofu slices in the hot sauce and cook 10 additional minutes.
4. Serve the tofu topped with plenty of sauce and chopped cilantro.

Chickpea Dip – Nohut Esmezi

Chickpeas are healthy, nutritious and filling, and this dip is exactly the same. Similar to a hummus, this chickpea dip uses pine nuts instead of tahini paste, so it has a nuttier flavor and a chunkier consistency.

Time: 20 minutes
Servings: 4-6

Ingredients:

   1 large can chickpeas, drained
   ¼ cup olive oil
   2 tablespoons lemon juice
   2 tablespoons pine nuts
   1 garlic clove
   Salt and pepper for taste

Directions:

1. Combine all the ingredients in a blender or food processor and pulse until smooth.
2. Adjust the taste with salt and pepper.
3. Spoon the dip in a serving bowl and serve it fresh.

Carrot Fritters

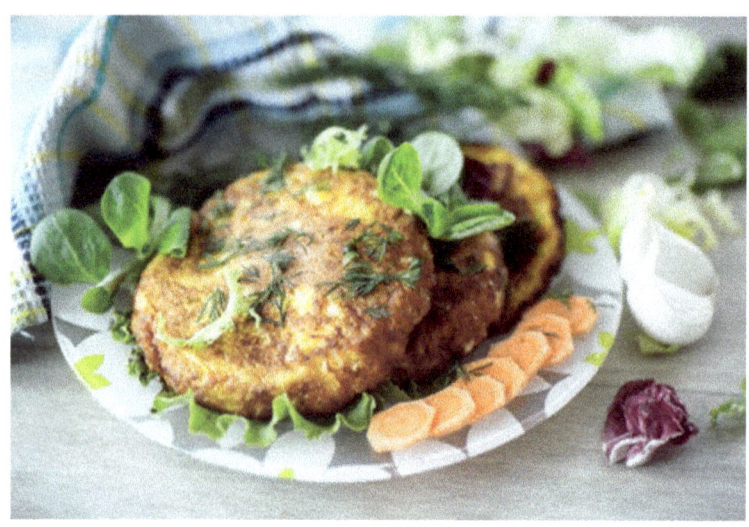

Turks are extremely inventive with their food. They often use ingredients that are easy to find that creates delicious dishes, like these carrot fritters.

Time: 35 minutes
Servings: 4-6

Ingredients:

   4 large carrots, grated
   ¼ cup black olives, pitted and chopped
   ½ cup chickpea flour
   2 tablespoons ground flaxseeds
   2 tablespoons water
   Salt and pepper for taste
   ½ teaspoon cumin powder
   1 pinch chili powder
   Oil for frying

Directions:

1. Combine all the ingredients in a bowl and mix well, seasoning with salt and pepper for taste.

2. Heat a few tablespoons of oil in a skillet then spoon the mixture into the hot oil.
3. Fry on each side for 2-3 minutes until golden brown then remove on paper towels.
4. Serve the fritters warm.

Spiced Cashew and Red Pepper Hummus

This hummus is not the classic, simple chickpea. Instead, it uses cashew nuts and roasted red peppers to create a rich and creamy dip, perfect with toasted bread or vegetable sticks.

Time: 20 minutes
Servings: 4-6

Ingredients:

   1 can chickpeas, drained
   4 roasted red bell peppers
   1 cup cashew nuts, soaked overnight
   3 tablespoons lemon juice
   1 garlic clove
   2 tablespoons tahini paste
   ½ teaspoon cayenne peppers
   Salt and pepper for taste

Directions:

   1. Combine all the ingredients in a blender or food processor.
   2. Pulse until smooth then adjust the taste with salt and pepper.
   3. Serve the hummus fresh.

Traditional Turkish Hummus

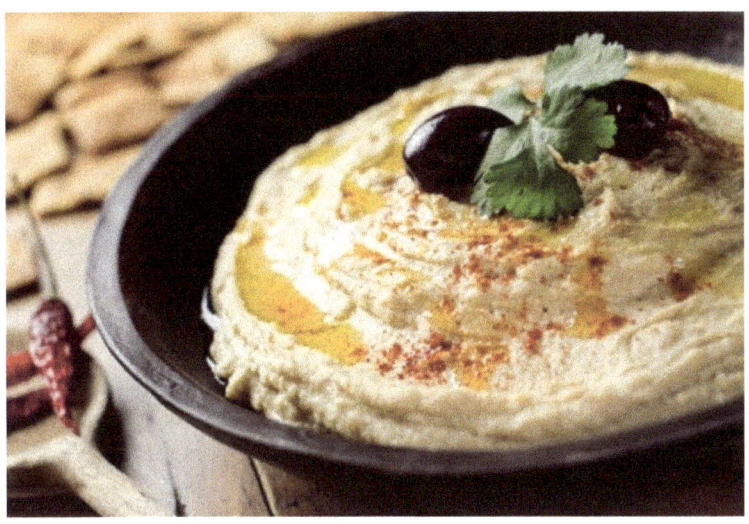

This recipe yields exactly the type of hummus you'd expect at a Turkish restaurant. It's rich, creamy and filling, perfect with flat bread.

Time: 20 minutes
Servings: 4-6

Ingredients:

  1 can chickpeas, drained
  ¼ cup tahini paste
  3 garlic cloves
  1 lemon, juiced
  Salt and pepper for taste
  ½ cup extra virgin olive oil

Directions:

1. Mix the chickpeas, tahini paste, garlic and lemon juice in a food processor.
2. Pulse until smooth, then gradually drizzle in half of the olive oil, mixing well.

3. Spoon the hummus into a serving bowl and top it with the remaining olive oil.
4. Serve the hummus fresh.

Tabbouleh Salad

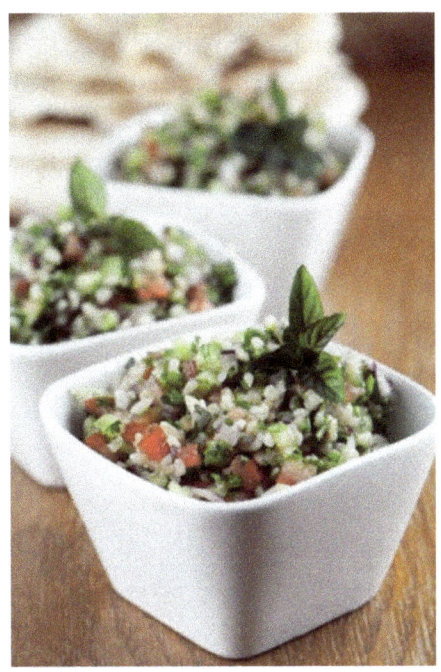

Tabbouleh salad is traditional for the Oriental area. But that's ok because it tastes amazing. It's incredibly refreshing and highly nutritious, so it's well worth a try!

Time: 30 minutes
Servings: 4-6

Ingredients:

2/3 cup bulgur, rinsed
1 cup hot water
4 green onions, sliced
1 cup chopped parsley
2 ripe tomatoes, sliced
1 lemon, juiced
Salt and pepper for taste
3 tablespoons olive oil

1. Mix the bulgur with hot water and let it soak up for 15 minutes or until all the liquid has been absorbed.
2. Stir in the remaining ingredients and mix gently.
3. Adjust the taste with salt and pepper if needed and serve the salad as fresh as possible.

Turkish Wedding Pilaf – Dugun Pilav

Pilaf is a rice dish, and it's incredibly versatile. It can be made either savory or sweet, and it's filling and nutritious which is why the Turkish prefer it. This wedding version is simple, but it shines!

Time: 40 minutes
Servings: 4-6

Ingredients:

  1 cup long grain rice, rinsed
  3 cups vegetable stock
  2 tablespoons olive oil
  1 carrot, cut into sticks
  ¼ cup pine nuts
  Salt and pepper for taste

Directions:

1. Mix the rice, stock, olive oil and carrot in a heavy saucepan.
2. Cook over low heat for 25 minutes or until most of the liquid has been absorbed.
3. Stir in the pine nuts, salt and pepper, and serve the pilaf warm.

Roasted Red Onions with Pomegranate Dressing

Roasting onions releases their natural sweetness, so this appetizer becomes incredibly tasty even though it only has a few basic ingredients.

Time: 30 minutes
Servings: 2-4

Ingredients:

6 red onions, quartered
Salt and pepper for taste
¼ cup olive oil
2 tablespoons pomegranate syrup
2 tablespoons balsamic vinegar

Directions:

1. Spread the onions in a baking tray and drizzle them with olive oil.
2. Season with salt and pepper and cook in the preheated oven at 400°F for 25 minutes or until slightly golden brown.
3. Mix the pomegranate syrup with balsamic vinegar. Then drizzle it over the roasted onions.
4. Serve the onions warm or chilled.

Brussel Sprouts and Pepper Appetizer

You'll see this kind of appetizers quite a lot in Turkish cuisine. They are a staple of the region and can be made with different vegetables as well.

Time: 45 minutes
Servings: 4-6

Ingredients:

16 oz. Brussel sprouts, halved
2 tablespoons olive oil
1 cup pearl onions
2 garlic cloves, chopped
1 cup crushed tomatoes
1 teaspoon smoked paprika
1 green pepper, sliced
2 tablespoons tomato paste
3 cups water
Salt and pepper for taste

Directions:

1. Pour water in a pot and bring it to a boil with a pinch of salt.
2. Throw in the sprouts and cook them for 5 minutes. Drain them well.
3. Heat the oil in a skillet and stir in the onions and garlic.
4. Sauté for 5 minutes then add the tomatoes, paprika, pepper and tomato paste.
5. Bring the sauce to a boil then add the sprouts.
6. Cook 10 additional minutes just until the sauce is reduced and thickened.
7. Adjust the taste with salt and pepper and serve the appetizer chilled.

Tomato and Onion Salad with Sumac Dressing – Gavurdagi Salad

Tomatoes and onions are a staple of Mediterranean cuisine, and Turkey sure finds inspiration in that. This salad shows how a simple recipe made with good quality ingredients beats any complex, exquisite recipe.

Time: 20 minutes
Servings: 2-4

Ingredients:

  1 red onion, sliced
  4 ripe tomatoes, sliced
  1 green pepper, sliced
  ¼ cup chopped parsley
  1 teaspoon sumac
  1 tablespoon balsamic vinegar
  3 tablespoons olive oil
  Salt and pepper for taste
  ¼ cup walnuts, chopped

Directions:

1. Mix the red onion, tomatoes, pepper and parsley in a salad bowl.
2. Combine the sumac, vinegar and olive oil in a separate bowl then drizzle this dressing over the salad.
3. Adjust the taste with salt and top with chopped walnuts.
4. Serve the salad as fresh as possible.

Eggplant Couscous Salad

This couscous salad is slightly smoky due to the grilled eggplant, but at the same time refreshing thanks to adding parsley and lemon juice. Bottom line is that it's a filling and nutritious salad, perfect as an appetizer as it tastes better chilled.

Time: 40 minutes
Servings: 4-6

Ingredients:

1 large eggplant, peeled and sliced
2 tablespoons olive oil
¾ cup couscous
1½ cups hot vegetable stock
½ cup chopped parsley
2 green onions, sliced
4 mint leaves, chopped
½ lemon, juiced
Salt and pepper for taste

Directions:

1. Brush the eggplant slices with olive oil.
2. Heat a grill pan over medium flame, then place the eggplant on the grill and cook on each side until golden brown.
3. Remove the eggplant and place in a bowl.
4. Mix the couscous with the hot stock in a bowl and let it soak up for 15 minutes.
5. Stir in the grilled eggplant, parsley, mint, green onions and lemon juice. Then adjust the taste with salt and pepper.
6. Mix gently and serve the salad chilled.

Spinach Phyllo Pie

This spinach pie can be found in most Turkish pastry shops at the savory section. It's made with layers of phyllo sheets and a delicious, garlicky spinach filling. Then it's cut into squares and served chilled.

Time: 1½ hours
Servings: 6-8

Ingredients:

    1 package phyllo dough sheets
    2 pounds fresh spinach, shredded
    4 tablespoons olive oil
    4 garlic cloves, minced
    1 shallot, chopped
    Salt and pepper for taste
    ½ teaspoon cumin powder
    ½ cup chopped cilantro
    ¼ cup olive oil for brushing the dough

Directions:

1. Heat 4 tablespoons olive oil in a skillet and stir in the garlic and shallot.
2. Sauté for 5 minutes, then stir in the spinach and cook for 15 minutes or until most of the liquid has evaporated.
3. Remove from heat and adjust the taste with salt, pepper, cumin and chopped cilantro.
4. Let the filling cool down for a few minutes.
5. Take a square pan and line its bottom with a few phyllo sheets.
6. Brush the dough with olive oil. Then spoon half of the spinach filling.
7. Top with a few more phyllo dough sheets and brush with olive oil again.
8. Top with the remaining phyllo dough sheets and brush with olive oil.

9. Cook in the preheated oven at 350°F for 35 minutes or until the top is golden brown and crisp.
10. Let the pie cool completely then cut into small squares.

Avokado Ezmesi – Avocado Dip

Similar to guacamole, this dip is rich and loaded with healthy ingredients, from avocado to herbs to tomatoes and lemon juice.

Time: 20 minutes
Servings: 2-4

Ingredients:

1 ripe avocado, mashed
2 tablespoons lemon juice
2 tablespoons coconut cream
1 cucumber, diced
2 ripe tomatoes, diced
2 garlic cloves, minced
1 small shallot, finely chopped
¼ cup chopped parsley
Salt and pepper for taste

Directions:

1. Combine all the ingredients in a bowl and mix well.
2. Season with salt and pepper for taste and serve the dip fresh.
3. To serve it, I recommend spooning it into a serving bowl. Place the bowl on a large platter and arrange flat breads, chips or vegetable sticks around it.

Eggplant Caviar

This eggplant caviar is basically a dip, but it tastes so good that it had to be called caviar!

Time: 1 hour
Servings: 4-6

Ingredients:

2 large eggplants, cut in half lengthwise
2 garlic cloves, minced
2 tablespoons lemon juice
¼ cup coconut cream
Salt and pepper for taste

Directions:

1. Place the eggplant halves in a baking tray and roast in the preheated oven at 375°F for 30 minutes.
2. When done, spoon the flesh of the eggplant in a bowl and mash it well with a fork.
3. Let the eggplant cool completely. Then stir in the garlic, lemon juice and coconut cream.
4. Add salt and pepper for taste and serve the caviar with flat bread.

Turkish Cucumber Dip

This dip is incredibly refreshing, and it's best served chilled. It's also very easy to make, and it will be ready in just under 10 minutes from start to finish.

Time: 10 minutes
Servings: 2-4

Ingredients:

2 seedless cucumbers, peeled
2 tablespoons chopped dill
1 cup cashew nuts, soaked overnight
2 tablespoons olive oil
Salt and pepper for taste
½ teaspoon lemon juice

Directions:

1. Combine all the ingredients in a blender or food processor and pulse until smooth.
2. Season the dip with salt and pepper and serve it as fresh as possible.

Chickpea Salad in Pita Pockets

Pita breads are so versatile! They can be served with pretty much anything, but here is a recipe that uses them differently. Since they rise and puff up during baking, a pocket is formed on the inside and guess what? You can stuff that pocket with salads or various fillings.

Time: 30 minutes
Servings: 6

Ingredients:

6 small pita breads
1 can chickpeas, drained
½ cup chopped parsley
2 ripe tomatoes, diced
1 cucumber, diced
1 red pepper, chopped
1 teaspoon cumin seeds
½ teaspoon coriander seeds
Salt and pepper for taste
2 tablespoons lemon juice

Directions:

1. Mix the chickpeas, parsley, tomatoes, cucumber, red pepper, cumin seeds, coriander seeds and lemon juice in a bowl.
2. Add salt and pepper for taste.
3. Carefully cut the top of each pita bread and reveal the pocket, the hole inside of the bread.
4. Stuff the pita breads with chickpea salad and serve them fresh.

SOUPS

Herbed Potato Soup

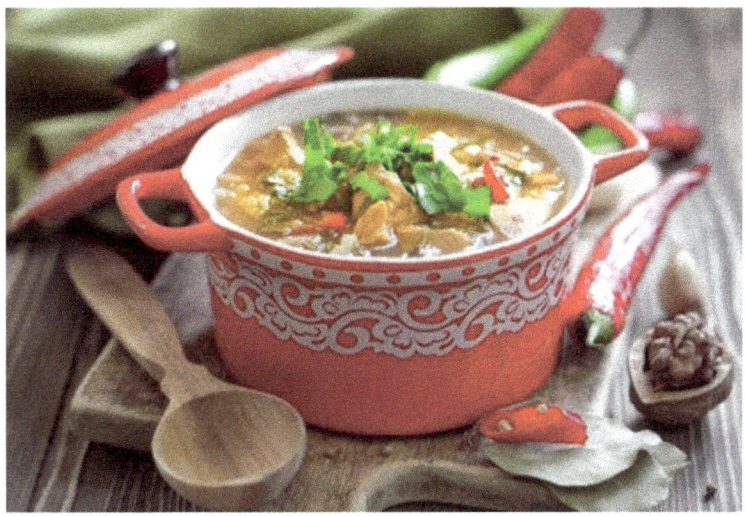

Nothing compares to a bowl of warm, hearty potato soup! It's comfort food at its best!

Time: 45 minutes
Servings: 4-6

Ingredients:

4 red potatoes, peeled and cubed
2 tablespoons olive oil
1 small onion, chopped
1 garlic clove, chopped
1 large carrot, diced
1 yellow bell pepper, cored and diced
2 ripe tomatoes, diced
2 cups vegetable stock
3 cups water

Salt and pepper for taste
3 tablespoons lemon juice
¼ cup chopped herbs of your choice

Directions:

1. Heat the oil in a soup pot and stir in the shallot, garlic, carrot and bell pepper.
2. Sauté for 2 minutes then add the potatoes, as well as stock, tomatoes, water, salt and pepper.
3. Cook the soup on medium flame for 30 minutes.
4. When done, remove from heat and stir in the lemon juice and herbs.
5. Serve the soup warm.

Vegetable Soup

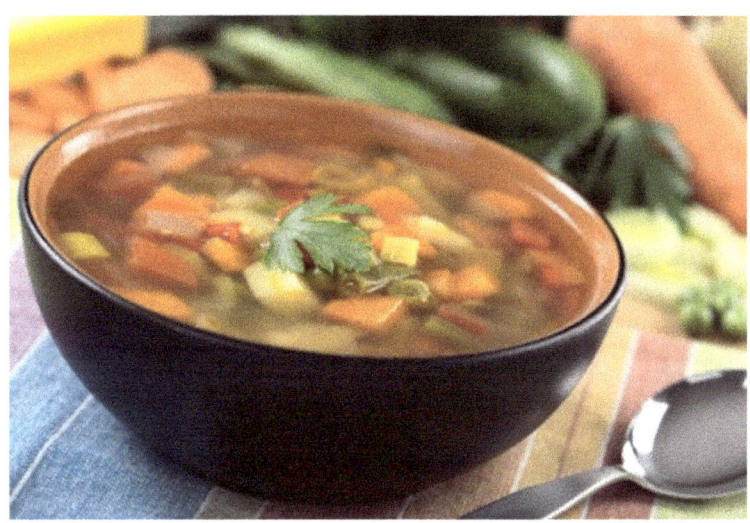

This soup is one of the most basic recipes there is, but it's healthy and comforting, especially during the cold season!

Time: 45 minutes
Servings: 6-8

Ingredients:

3 tablespoons olive oil
1 sweet onion, chopped
1 red bell pepper, cored and pepper
1 large carrot, diced
1 zucchini, cubed
2 red potatoes, peeled and cubed
2 tablespoons white rice, rinsed
6 cups water
Salt and pepper for taste
1 tablespoon chopped parsley

Directions:

1. Heat the olive oil in a soup pot and stir in the onion, bell pepper and carrot.

2. Sauté for 2 minutes then stir in the zucchini, potatoes, rice and water.
3. Add salt and pepper for taste and cook over medium flame for 30 minutes.
4. Serve the soup warm, topped with chopped parsley.

Beetroot Cabbage Soup – Kafkas Corbasi

This earthy soup is so comforting in the cold season! And healthy as well, considering the fact that the beetroot is a bomb of antioxidants and vitamins.

Time: 45 minutes
Servings: 4-6

Ingredients:

2 tablespoons olive oil
1 red onion, chopped
½ celery stalk, sliced
2 carrots, diced
1 beetroot, peeled and grated
½ head cabbage, shredded
4 cups water
Salt and pepper for taste
2 tablespoons chopped cilantro

Directions:

1. Heat the olive oil in a soup pot and stir in the red onion, celery and carrots.
2. Sauté for 5 minutes then stir in the beetroot, cabbage, water, salt and pepper.
3. Cook the soup over medium flame for 30 minutes.
4. Serve the soup warm, topped with chopped cilantro.

Vegan Sultan's Soup

This soup is an interpretation of a meaty soup called Sultan's Soup. It is light and delicious, despite its name which might make you think it is rich and loaded with luxurious ingredients.

Time: 50 minutes
Servings: 4-6

Ingredients:

6 oz. firm tofu, cubed
2 tablespoons olive oil
3 tablespoons all-purpose flour
1½ cups almond milk
3 cups vegetable stock
¼ cup ground almonds
Salt and pepper for taste
1 pinch nutmeg

Directions:

1. Heat the olive oil in a soup pot and stir in the flour. Cook for 1 minute then add almond milk and cook until thickened.
2. Add the stock, tofu and almonds as well as salt and pepper.
3. Cook the soup for 15 minutes on low heat.
4. When done, remove from heat and stir in the nutmeg.
5. Serve the soup warm.

Red Lentil and Bulgur Soup – Ezogelin

Ezogelin soup is also known as the Bride's soup. It's made with lentils, bulgur and rice. It's rich and filling.

Time: 50 minutes
Servings: 4-6

Ingredients:

4 tablespoons olive oil
1 onion, chopped
1 cup red lentils
½ cup coarse bulgur
4 cups water
2 cups vegetable stock
½ cup tomato sauce
Salt and pepper for taste
1 bay leaf
2 tablespoons chopped parsley

Directions:

1. Heat the olive oil in a soup pot and stir in the onion. Sauté for 2 minutes.
2. Stir in the red lentils and bulgur. Then add the water, stock and tomato sauce.
3. Add the bay leaf, salt and pepper and cook the soup for 30 minutes.
4. Serve the soup warm, topped with chopped parsley.

Creamy Lentil Soup

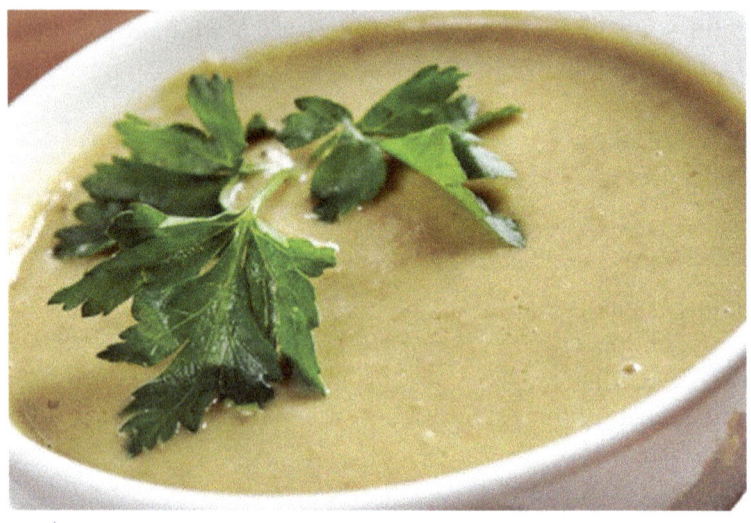

Lentils are quite common in Turkish cuisine because not only they taste great, but they are also filling and nutritious. Plus, they make an excellent creamy soup!

Time: 40 minutes
Servings: 6-8

Ingredients:

   3 tablespoons olive oil
   2 onions, chopped
   1 teaspoon hot paprika
   1½ cups red lentils
   2 tablespoons tomato paste
   7 cups vegetable stock
   1 teaspoon dried mint
   2 tablespoons lemon juice
   Salt and pepper for taste

Directions:

1. Heat the olive oil in a soup pot and stir in the onion. Cook for 5 minutes until soft and translucent.

2. Add paprika, lentils, tomato paste and stock, as well as mint, salt and pepper.
3. Cook the soup on medium flame for 30 minutes. Stir in the lemon juice.
4. When done, puree the soup with an immersion blender and serve it as fresh as possible.

Bean and Lentil Soup with Sumac

Sumac is a tangy seasoning specific to the Oriental zone, and it really makes this soup shine!

Time: 45 minutes
Servings: 4-6

Ingredients:

2 tablespoons olive oil
1 shallot, chopped
2 garlic cloves, chopped
1 carrot, diced
1 can black beans, drained
¾ cup red lentils, rinsed
5 cups water
½ cup tomato sauce
Salt and pepper for taste
1 tablespoon sumac

Directions:

1. Heat the oil in a soup pot and stir in the shallot and garlic. Sauté for 1 minute then add the carrot, black beans and lentils.
2. Stir in the water and tomato sauce as well as salt and pepper.
3. Cook the soup on medium flame for 25 minutes.
4. When done, remove from heat and stir in the sumac.
5. Serve the soup warm.

Vegetable and Rice Soup

Based on a vegetable stock, this soup may look simple, but its taste is comforting and great for those days when you're struggling with a cold.

Time: 1 hour
Servings: 4-6

Ingredients:

1 onion, halved
2 red bell peppers, cored and sliced
2 carrots, sliced
2 celery stalks, sliced
2 garlic cloves, whole
7 cups water
Salt and pepper for taste
3/4 cup rice, rinsed

Directions:

1. Combine the onion, bell peppers, carrots, celery, garlic and water in a soup pot.
2. Add salt and pepper for taste and cook the soup on low heat for 30 minutes.
3. When done, remove and discard the vegetables, or use them for a different dish.
4. Place the soup back on heat and stir in the rice.
5. Cook for 15 additional minutes.
6. Serve the soup warm.

Rustic Soup

The highlight of this soup is the incredible taste given by the caraway seeds!

Time: 45 minutes
Servings: 8-10

Ingredients:

4 tablespoons olive oil
1 onion, chopped
2 large carrots, diced
2 celery stalk, sliced
2 garlic cloves, chopped
2 cups shredded cabbage
1½ teaspoons caraways seeds
1 can diced tomatoes
6 cups water
Salt and pepper for taste
6 oz. one-day old bread, cubed

Directions:

1. Heat the oil in a soup pot and stir in the onion, carrots, celery and garlic.
2. Sauté for 2 minutes then stir in the cabbage, caraways seeds, tomatoes and water and cook the soup for 20 minutes.
3. Adjust the taste with salt and pepper. Then remove the soup from heat and stir in the bread cubes.
4. Serve the soup warm.

Winter Soup

Needless to say that this soup is made generally during the cold season, for it's made with bulgur and plenty of Turkish spices.

Time: 1 hour
Servings: 6-8

Ingredients:

2 tablespoons olive oil
2 leeks, sliced
2 carrots, diced
2 parsnips, diced
2 garlic cloves, chopped
½ teaspoon cumin seeds
¼ teaspoon coriander seeds
1 teaspoon dried mint
2 tablespoons tomato paste
8 cups water
1 can chickpeas, drained
¾ cup bulgur, rinsed
Salt and pepper for taste

Directions:

1. Heat the olive oil in a soup pot and stir in the leeks and garlic.
2. Sauté for 2 minutes then add the carrots, parsnips, cumin seeds, coriander seeds, mint and tomato paste. Sauté for 5 minutes.
3. Add the water, chickpeas and bulgur, as well as salt and pepper for taste. Cook for 30 minutes.
4. Serve the soup warm.

Creamy Pumpkin Soup with Cumin Dressing

The highlight of this soup is the cumin dressing which infuses the soup in such a delicious manner!

Time: 50 minutes
Servings: 4-6

Ingredients:

4 cups pumpkin cubes
1 tablespoon olive oil
1 sweet onion, chopped
1 garlic clove, minced
1 teaspoon paprika
1 teaspoon mustard seeds
4 cups vegetable stock
Salt and pepper for taste
2 tablespoons olive oil
1 teaspoon cumin seeds
1 teaspoon coriander seeds

Directions:

1. Heat 1 tablespoon olive oil in a soup pot and stir in the shallot and garlic. Sauté for 2 minutes then add the pumpkin, paprika, mustard seeds and stock.
2. Add salt and pepper for taste and cook the soup for 30 minutes.
3. When done, puree the soup with an immersion blender.
4. For the dressing, heat the oil in a small skillet. Add the cumin seeds and coriander seeds and sauté for 2 minutes just until they begin to pop.
5. Pour the soup in serving bowls and drizzle with the cumin dressing.
6. Serve the soup warm.

MAIN DISHES

Cracked Wheat Pilaf

Wheat is a great replacer for rice, and they have a similar nutritional profile. Wheat tastes nuttier though, and it's fairly common in Turkey or surrounding countries.

Time: 45 minutes
Servings: 4-6

Ingredients:

2 tablespoons olive oil
1 sweet onion, chopped
2/3 cup cracked wheat
½ cup bulgur
3 cups vegetable stock
1 can diced tomatoes
Salt and pepper for taste

Directions:

1. Heat the oil in a heavy saucepan and stir in the onion. Sauté until soft and translucent.
2. Stir in the wheat and bulgur and cook them for 2 additional minutes.
3. Add the stock and tomatoes, then season with salt and pepper and cook on low to medium flame for 30 minutes.
4. Serve the pilaf warm.

Imam Baialdi – Stuffed Eggplants

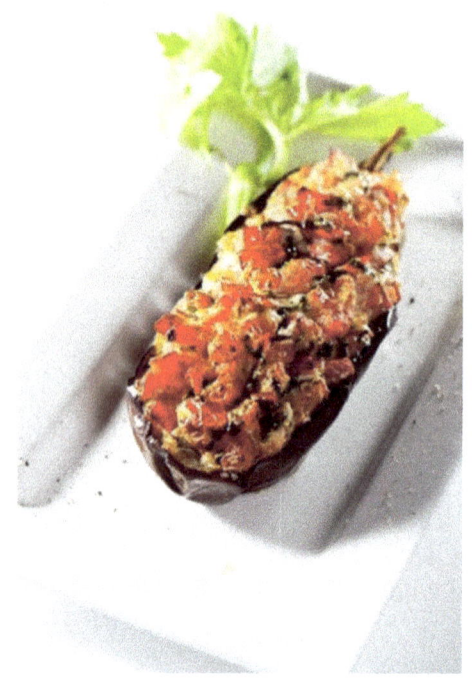

Imam Baialdi is a dish that doesn't need any introduction, for it is known worldwide. In my opinion it's a dish that proves the versatility and deliciousness of eggplants.

Time: 1 hour
Servings: 4

Ingredients:

2 large eggplants
2 tablespoons olive oil
1 red onion, finely chopped
2 garlic cloves, minced
4 oz. firm tofu, crumbled
½ teaspoon mustard seeds
½ teaspoon cumin powder
2 ripe tomatoes, diced
Salt and pepper for taste

Directions:

1. Cut the eggplants in half lengthwise and carefully remove the flesh with a spoon, leaving the skins intact.
2. Chop the flesh finely.
3. Heat the oil in a skillet and stir in the red onion. Sauté for 2 minutes then add the eggplant flesh as well as tofu, mustard seeds, cumin powder and tomatoes.
4. Season with salt and pepper and cook on medium flame for 10 minutes.
5. Spoon the mixture into the eggplant skins and cook in the preheated oven at 350°F for 20 minutes.
6. Serve the imam baialdi warm.

Eggplant and Tomato Towers

These vegetable towers look incredibly festive and taste amazing when served with a balsamic dressing.

Time: 40 minutes
Servings: 4-6

Ingredients:

1 large eggplant, finely sliced
2 tablespoons olive oil
2 large ripe tomatoes, sliced
2 tablespoons balsamic vinegar
1 tablespoon lemon juice
1 tablespoon Dijon mustard
Salt and pepper for taste

Directions:

1. Brush the eggplant slices with olive oil.
2. Heat a grill pan over medium flame then place the eggplant slices on the grill and cook on each side until browned.
3. When done, layer the eggplant slices and tomato slices on a serving plate.
4. For the dressing, mix the balsamic vinegar with lemon juice and mustard, as well as salt and pepper.
5. Drizzle the towers with the dressing and serve them fresh.

Prasa Yahnisi – Turkish Stewed Leeks

Similar to the braised leeks, this recipe is mainly made of leeks and tomatoes. It is as simple as this sounds. Let me tell you that it tastes amazing, and it's a great way of adding variety to your vegan day-to-day menus.

Time: 40 minutes
Servings: 2-4

Ingredients:

2 pounds leeks, cut into 2-inch pieces
4 tablespoons olive oil
2 red onions, chopped
4 ripe tomatoes, peeled and chopped
1 cup vegetable stock
Salt and pepper for taste
1 bay leaf
½ teaspoon cumin seeds

Directions:

1. Heat the olive oil in a saucepan and stir in the onions. Sauté for 5 minutes then add the tomatoes, stock, bay leaf, cumin seeds, salt and pepper.
2. Bring the sauce to a boil then stir in the leeks.
3. Cover with a lid and stew on low heat for 30 minutes.
4. Serve the dish warm.

Turkish Rice Casserole

Rice is a basic food encountered in many cuisines. Turkish cook rice in many ways, but their favorite has to be pilaf or this casserole which is similar to pilaf, but it's easier to make.

Time: 1 hour
Servings: 6-8

Ingredients:

2 cups long grain rice, rinsed
½ teaspoon turmeric powder
½ teaspoon cumin seeds
2 ripe tomatoes, chopped
1 cup green peas
½ cup raisins
1 cup chopped pistachio
3 cups vegetable stock
Salt and pepper for taste

Directions:

1. Combine all the ingredients in a deep dish baking pan.
2. Add salt and pepper for taste and cover the pan with an aluminum foil.
3. Cook in the preheated oven at 330°F for 45 minutes.
4. Serve the casserole warm.

Spiced Tofu Kabobs

Kabobs are traditional for Turkey. Even though the traditional ones are made with lamb meat, here is a version that uses tofu as a replacer. Feel free to use mushrooms if you're not a huge fan of tofu.

Time: 50 minutes
Servings: 4-6

Ingredients:

10 oz. firm tofu, cubed
1 teaspoon cumin powder
½ teaspoon sumac
2 tablespoons olive oil
1 cup cherry tomatoes
1 cup pearl onions

Directions:

1. Season the tofu with cumin powder and sumac. Then drizzle them with olive oil.
2. Layer the tofu, tomatoes and pearl onions on wooden skewers.
3. Heat a grill pan over medium flame then place the kabobs on the hot grill.
4. Cook on each side for 2 minutes or until golden brown and serve the kabobs warm.

Grilled Portobello Kabobs

Portobello mushrooms are amazing, for they have a high content of protein, and their nutritional profile makes them similar to meat. They become a vegan's meat and one of the main sources of iron and proteins.

Time: 40 minutes
Servings: 4-6

Ingredients:

4 Portobello mushrooms, quartered
2 red onions, sliced
2 red bell peppers, cored and cubed
Salt and pepper for taste
3 tablespoons olive oil

Directions:

1. Layer the mushrooms, onions and bell peppers on wooden skewers.
2. Season with salt and pepper and drizzle with olive oil.
3. Heat a grill pan over medium flame and place the kabobs on the hot grill. Cook for 2-3 minutes on each side.
4. Serve the kabobs warm.

Tofu Burgers

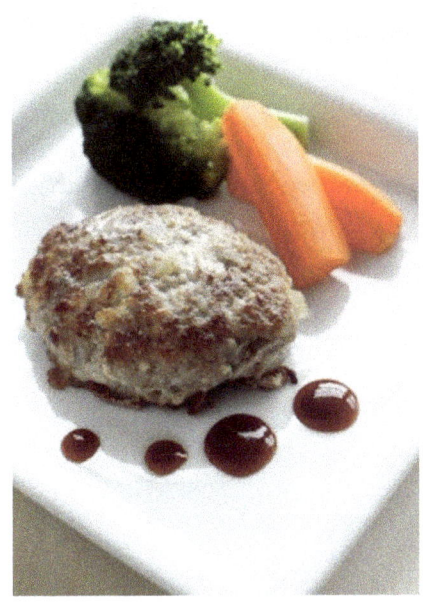

You don't need to give up on burgers once you go vegan! A burger made with vegan ingredients is just as juicy and delicious!

Time: 40 minutes
Servings: 4-6

Ingredients:

   10 oz. silken tofu
   2 tablespoons olive oil
   1 shallot, chopped
   2 garlic cloves, minced
   ½ teaspoon cumin powder
   ½ teaspoon paprika
   1 teaspoon ground turmeric
   1 cup prepared hummus
   1 cup breadcrumbs
   Salt and pepper for taste
   3 tablespoons vegetable oil for frying

Directions:

1. Mix the tofu, olive oil, shallot, garlic, cumin, paprika, turmeric, hummus and breadcrumbs in a food processor.
2. Pulse just until mixed.
3. Wet your hands and form small burger patties.
4. Heat the oil in a skillet and place the burgers in the hot oil.
5. Fry on each side until golden brown and crusty. Serve the burgers warm in burger buns with your favorite topping.

Eggplants Stuffed with Chickpeas

This vegan dish is packed with great textures and flavors – nutty chickpeas, earthy walnuts and refreshing parsley.

Time: 1 hour
Servings: 4

Ingredients:

2 large eggplants cut in half lengthwise
1 cup canned chickpeas, drained
1 red chili, chopped
½ teaspoon cumin seeds
1 ripe tomato, diced
2 tablespoons lemon juice
Salt and pepper for taste
½ cup chopped walnuts

Directions:

1. Carefully remove the flesh of the chickpeas and chop it finely.
2. Mix the eggplant flesh with chickpeas, chili, cumin seeds, tomato, lemon juice salt and pepper in a bowl.
3. Spoon the filling into the eggplant skins and top with chopped walnuts.
4. Cook in the preheated oven at 350°F for 30 minutes or until the veggies turn soft.
5. Serve the stuffed eggplants warm.

Spicy Falafel

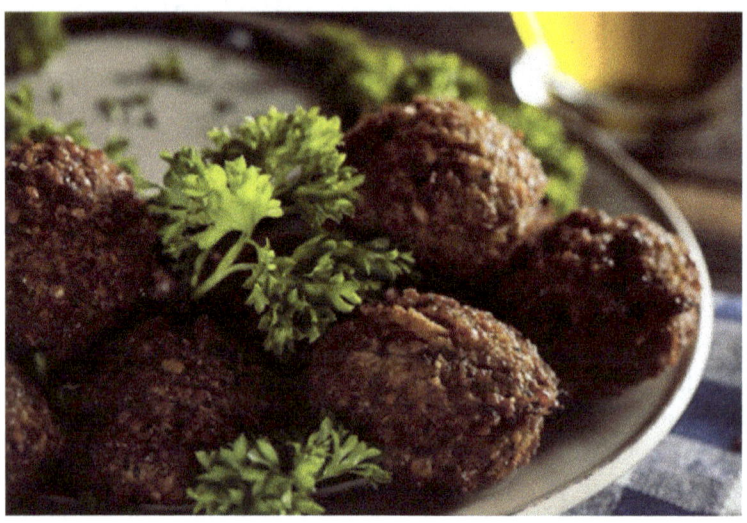

It's almost impossible that you've never heard of falafel before. It's a well-known chickpea dish and loved all around the world. But you can make it at home too! No need to drive to that Oriental takeaway.

Time: 1 hour
Servings: 6-8

Ingredients:

2 cans chickpeas, drained
1 sweet onion, finely chopped
1 teaspoon cumin powder
1 teaspoon ground cumin
2 garlic cloves, minced
2 tablespoons ground flax seeds
¼ cup chopped parsley
Salt and pepper for taste
2 cups vegetable oil for frying

1. Mix the chickpeas, onion, cumin powder, garlic, flax seeds, salt and pepper in a food processor and pulse until well combined and ground.
2. Stir in the parsley then heat the oil in a deep frying pan.
3. Form small patties and drop them in the hot oil.
4. Fry the falafel on each side until golden brown and remove the patties on paper towels.
5. Serve the patties warm, alone or wrapped in flat bread with your favorite toppings.

Mushroom Stuffed Zucchini Boats

Don't underestimate this mild vegetable. The zucchini makes juicy, flavorful meals, and this recipe is the perfect example.

Time: 1 hour
Servings: 6

Ingredients:

3 large zucchinis
4 Portobello mushrooms
2 garlic cloves
1 shallot
¼ cup chopped parsley
1 teaspoon dried thyme
½ teaspoon dried mint
Salt and pepper for taste
1 can diced tomatoes

Directions:

1. Cut the zucchinis in half lengthwise and carefully remove the flesh with a spoon, leaving the skins intact.
2. Combine the zucchini flesh, mushrooms, garlic, shallot, parsley, thyme and mint in a food processor. Pulse just until ground, but not too fine.
3. Season with salt and pepper then spoon the mixture into the zucchini skins.
4. Spread the tomatoes on the bottom of a deep dish baking pan.
5. Place the zucchini boats in the pan as well and cook in the preheated oven at 350°F for 35 minutes.
6. Serve the zucchinis warm.

Turkish Eggplant and Squash Bake

Similar to a ratatouille, this bake is so flavorful that you will ask for a second portion. It's incredibly healthy as well!

Time: 1 hour
Servings: 6-8

Ingredients:

2 eggplants, peeled and cubed
2 cups butternut squash cubes
2 red onions, quartered
1 teaspoon cumin seeds
1 teaspoon coriander seeds
1 teaspoon mustard seeds
1 teaspoon turmeric powder
4 tablespoons olive oil
1 tablespoon dried herbs (thyme, oregano, sage)
Salt and pepper for taste

Directions:

1. Combine all the ingredients in a deep baking pan and mix to evenly distribute them.
2. Season with salt and pepper as needed and cook in the preheated oven at 350°F for 35 minutes.
3. Serve the bake warm.

Grilled Eggplant with Hummus

Grilled eggplant slices are spread with hummus and topped with walnuts for this filling and rich main dish. And they make up such a nutritious meal!

Time: 30 minutes
Servings: 6

Ingredients:

1 large eggplant, sliced
2 tablespoons olive oil
Salt and pepper for taste
10 oz. prepared hummus
½ cup chopped walnuts
1 teaspoon dried mint
¼ teaspoon chili flakes

Directions:

1. Brush the eggplant slices with olive oil then season them with salt and pepper.
2. Heat a grill pan over medium flame and place the eggplant on the grill.
3. Cook them on each side for 2-3 minutes or until browned.
4. When done, remove the eggplant on a plate and spread the hummus over each slice.
5. Top each eggplant slice with walnuts, mint and a touch of chili flakes.
6. Serve the eggplant slices fresh.

Stuffed Artichokes

Fresh artichokes are hard to clean and peel, but they are worth the task! What you get in the end is a filling, rich, nutritious meal, perfect for lunch or dinner, either warm or chilled.

Time: 1½ hours
Servings: 6

Ingredients:

6 large fresh artichokes
4 Portobello mushrooms, chopped
1 sweet onion, chopped
2 tablespoons olive oil
4 ripe tomatoes, chopped
½ cup white rice, rinsed
¼ cup chopped parsley
½ teaspoon cumin powder
½ teaspoon paprika
Salt and pepper for taste
3 cups water
1 lemon, juiced

Directions:

1. Carefully peel the artichokes and carve the center with the help of a spoon. Place them in water with lemon juice while peeling as they tend to oxidize quickly.
2. Heat the oil in a skillet and stir in the onion. Sauté for 2 minutes or until soft and translucent.
3. Stir in the tomatoes, rice, parsley, cumin powder, paprika, salt and pepper and cook until most of the liquid has evaporated.
4. Drain the artichokes and stuff them with the mushroom filling.
5. Place the artichokes with the cut facing up in a deep saucepan.
6. Pour in the water and cook for 40 minutes on medium heat, covered with a lid.
7. Serve the artichokes warm.

Spinach Filled Flatbreads

Flatbreads are a version of tortillas that can be stuffed with pretty much anything. This spinach version is one of the healthiest and most delicious versions.

Time: 30 minutes
Servings: 4

Ingredients:

2 tablespoons olive oil
1 sweet onion, sliced
1 pound baby spinach
½ teaspoon chili flakes
¼ teaspoon cumin powder
1 pinch nutmeg
Salt and pepper for taste
4 oz. firm tofu, crumbled
4 flatbreads

Directions:

1. Heat the oil in a skillet and stir in the onion. Sauté for 2 minutes until soft and translucent then add the spinach, chili flakes, cumin powder and nutmeg.
2. Cook for 10-15 minutes until most of the liquid evaporates then remove from heat and stir in the tofu.
3. Adjust the taste with salt and pepper if needed and spoon the filling into flatbreads.
4. Serve the wraps warm.

No Meat Meatballs

These no meat meatballs are juicy and incredibly flavorful for a dish that hasn't seen any meat.

Time: 1 hour
Servings: 4-6

Ingredients:

1 large sweet onion
2 garlic cloves
2 boiled potatoes
1 can lentils, drained
1 celery stalk
1 bunch parsley
2 tablespoons ground flax seeds
1 teaspoon cumin powder
1 teaspoon dried oregano
Salt and pepper for taste
4 tablespoons olive oil

Directions:

1. Combine all the ingredients in a food processor and pulse until well mixed.
2. Adjust the taste with salt and pepper if needed then wet your hands and form small balls.
3. Place them all on a baking tray lined with parchment paper and cook in the preheated oven at 350°F for 25 minutes.
4. Let them cool in the pan before serving.

DESSERTS

Asure – Wheat and Rice Pudding

Rice and wheat puddings are traditional for Turkish cuisine as they are easy to make and can take on a lot of flavors, from orange blossom to rose and with nutty touches.

Time: 45 minutes
Servings: 4-6

Ingredients:

  1 cup wheat
  1 cup rice
  ½ cup raisins
  ½ cup dried apricots, chopped
  1 cup sugar
  4 cups almond milk

Directions:

1. Combine the wheat, rice, raisins, apricots and almond milk in a heavy saucepan.
2. Cook over low heat for 35 minutes then stir in the sugar and remove from heat.
3. Pour the pudding into individual serving bowls and let it cool before serving.

Sari Burma Dessert

Sari burma is similar to Baklava, but it's shaped into a roll which is then baked and soaked into a rich sugar syrup. They take a while to make, but it's well worth the effort.

Time: 2 hours
Servings: 10

Ingredients:

   1 package phyllo dough sheets
   1 pound walnuts, ground
   ½ cup coconut oil
   2 cups sugar
   2 cups water
   1 teaspoon orange blossom water

Directions:

1. Take 2 sheets of phyllo dough and place them on your working surface.
2. Spread a few tablespoons of walnuts at one end then roll tightly.
3. Transfer the roll into a baking tray and repeat with the remaining dough sheets and walnuts.
4. Drizzle the dessert with coconut oil.
5. Bake the dessert in the preheated oven at 350°F for 30 minutes or until the top is golden brown and crisp.
6. In the meantime, make the syrup by boiling the water and sugar for 5 minutes.
7. Remove from heat and stir in the orange blossom water.
8. Pour the hot syrup over the dessert and let it soak up until it cools down.
9. Carefully cut into smaller pieces and serve it chilled.

Spiced squash

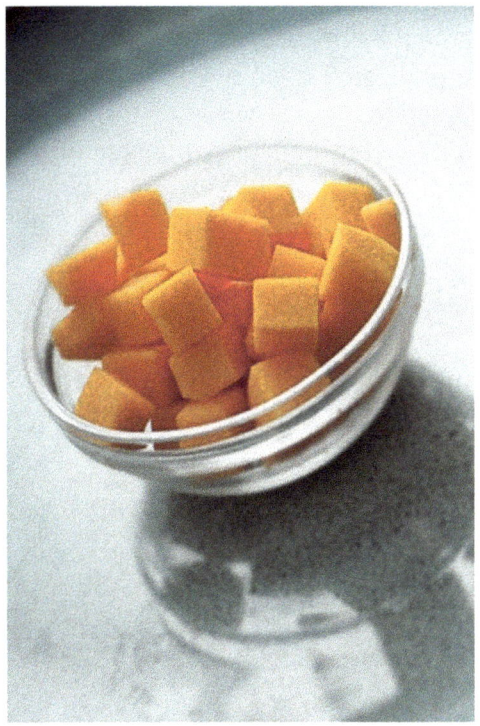

Every Turkish dessert includes spices in a way or another, but this squash dessert beats them all having cinnamon, cardamom, whole cloves and star anise.

Time: 1 hour
Servings: 6-8

Ingredients:

   5 cups cubed butternut squash
   1 teaspoon cinnamon powder
   1 teaspoon ground cardamom
   1 teaspoon ground star anise
   ¼ teaspoon ground black pepper
   ½ cup brown sugar

Directions:

1. Mix the squash cubes with the rest of the ingredients then spread them on a baking tray lined with parchment paper.
2. Bake in the preheated oven at 350°F for 40 minutes or until slightly caramelized.
3. Let them cool in the pan then transfer in a bowl and serve fresh.

Semolina and Dried Fruit Halva

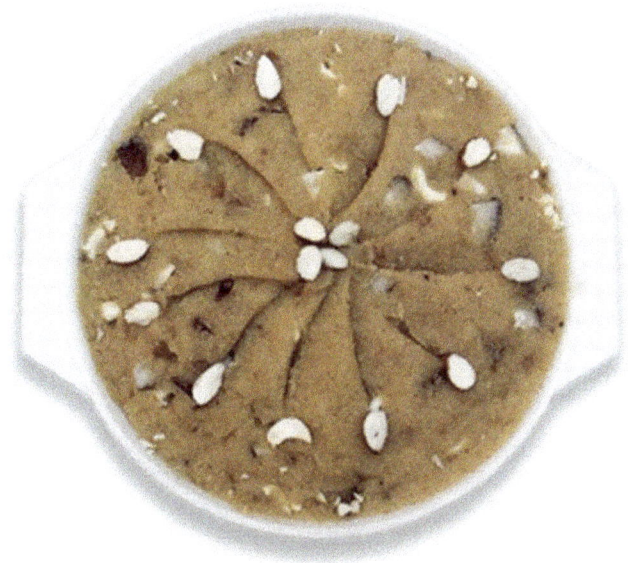

You will see plenty of dried fruits in Turkish desserts, but that's ok because dried fruits pack a lot of flavor and natural sweetness. They bring a flavor boost to every recipe using them.

Time: 40 minutes
Servings: 4-6

Ingredients:

¼ cup coconut oil
1½ cups medium semolina
1½ cups sugar
1 cup water
1½ cups almond milk
¼ cup raisins
¼ cup dried apricots, chopped

Directions:

1. Heat the coconut oil in a heavy saucepan.

2. Stir in the semolina and cook it for 5 minutes, stirring all the time, just until it becomes golden brown.
3. Pour in the water and almond milk, stirring all the time. Cook for 10 minutes, stirring all the time.
4. Stir in the sugar, raisins and apricots and remove from heat.
5. Pour the halva in individual serving bowls and let it cool completely.
6. When done, turn it upside down and serve it fresh.

Stewed Apricots

Although simple, this recipe is delightful. The dried apricots pack so much flavor and natural sweetness that this dessert barely needs any sweetener.

Time: 30 minutes
Servings: 2-4

Ingredients:

1 cup dried apricots
1 cup fresh orange juice
2 cups water
¼ cup sugar
1 cardamom pod, crushed
1 star anise

Directions:

1. Combine all the ingredients in a saucepan and bring to a boil.
2. Cover with a lid and cook for 20-30 minutes until the apricots become soft.
3. Remove from heat and serve them chilled.

Syrup Cookies

The highlight of these cookies is the fact that they are soaked in syrup after baking. This makes them moist and sweet, incredibly delicious.

Time: 1 hour
Servings: 2 dozen

Ingredients:

1 cup coconut oil
½ cup almond milk
½ cup sugar
1 tablespoon lemon zest
1 tablespoon lemon juice
1 teaspoon baking soda
½ teaspoon baking powder
1 pinch salt
3 cups all-purpose flour
2 cup sugar
2 cups water
1 teaspoon orange water

Directions:

1. To make the syrup, combine 2 cups of sugar with 2 cups of water and boil for 5 minutes. Remove from heat, and stir in the orange water then let it cool.
2. To make the cookies, combine all the ingredients in a food processor and pulse until a nice dough is obtained.
3. Grease your hands and form small balls.
4. Place all the balls on a baking tray lined with parchment paper. Then flatten them slightly with a fork.
5. Bake in the preheated oven at 350°F for 15-20 minutes or until slightly golden brown and crisp.
6. When done, remove from the pan and dip them quickly into the chilled sugar syrup. Don't let them soak up too much, for they will break. They only need to infuse slightly.
7. Serve the cookies fresh and chilled.

Gullac

This dessert is made once again with phyllo dough sheets which may be considered a staple of Turkish cuisine. It's a dessert that focuses on the flavor combination between almonds and rose water, and it's delicate and exquisite.

Time: 1 hour
Servings: 10-12

Ingredients:

  1 package phyllo dough sheets
  1 pound almonds, ground
  3 cups almond milk
  2 cups sugar
  2 teaspoons rose water

Directions:

1. Layer the phyllo dough sheets with ground almonds in a baking tray.
2. Bake in the preheated oven at 350°F for 30-40 minutes or until crisp and golden brown.
3. For the syrup, combine the almond milk with sugar in a saucepan and cook until all the sugar has been dissolved.
4. Remove the gullac from the oven and pour the syrup over the baked dessert.
5. Let it soak up and cut into small squares.
6. Serve chilled.

Noah's Ark Pudding

Legends say that this pudding is one of the first desserts ever made. Some people believe that Noah himself made it for the first time. True or not, this pudding is delicious and rich, a great example of how Turkish desserts are!

Time: 40 minutes
Servings: 6-8

Ingredients:

  3 cups barley, rinsed
  1 cup canned chickpeas, drained
  1 cup navy beans, rinsed and drained
  ¼ cup white rice, rinsed
  4 cups almond milk
  ¼ cup dried currants
  ¼ cup pine nuts
  ¼ cup dried apricots, chopped
  ¼ cup dried figs, chopped
  3 cups sugar
  1 cinnamon stick

Directions:

1. Combine the barley, chickpeas, beans and rice in a heavy saucepan and bring to a boil over medium flame.
2. Cook for 30 minutes, then add the remaining ingredients and cook for 10 additional minutes.
3. Spoon the pudding into individual serving bowls and let the pudding cool completely before serving.

Pumpkin Dessert with Tahini Sauce

Time: 1 hour
Servings: 4-6

Ingredients:

2 pounds pumpkin, peeled and cut into large cubes
1 cup dark brown sugar
1 teaspoon cinnamon powder
½ cup tahini paste
½ cup chopped walnuts

Directions:

1. Place the pumpkin cubes on a baking tray lined with parchment paper.
2. Sprinkle with brown sugar and cinnamon. Bake in the preheated oven at 350°F for 40 minutes.
3. When done, remove from the oven and let the pumpkin cool down.
4. Drizzle with tahini paste and sprinkle with walnuts just before serving.

Turkish Chocolate Halva

Halva is an Oriental dish known all over the world, but you can make your own version at home. It's simple to make, and you can customize it to fit your likings.

Time: 20 minutes
Servings: 4-6

Ingredients:

2 cups water
2 cups all-purpose flour
¼ cup cocoa powder
1 cup brown sugar
¼ cup coconut oil
½ cup chopped walnuts

Directions:

1. Bring the water and sugar to a boil in a heavy saucepan.
2. In a different saucepan, heat the oil then stir in the flour and cocoa powder.
3. Cook the flour for 2 minutes then pour in the hot water mixture.
4. Cook until it thickens so much that it forms a ball.
5. Stir in the walnuts then spoon the halva into small individual bowls and let it cool completely before serving.

Orange and Pistachio Turkish Delight

This delicious treat tastes like orange and pistachio and can now be made at home. No need to wonder how Turkish delight is made because now you know!

Time: 2 hours
Servings: 4 dozen

Ingredients:

1 pound white sugar
1 cup water
1 tablespoon lemon juice
1 cup cornstarch
½ teaspoon cream of tartar
1 cup water
2 teaspoons orange blossom water
½ cup pistachio, chopped

Directions:

1. Combine the sugar and water, as well as lemon juice in a heavy saucepan.
2. Place the saucepan over medium flame and bring to a boil. Cook the syrup until it reaches the soft ball stage, meaning that when you pour a few drops of syrup in a cup of cold water, you can gather the syrup into a soft bowl.
3. While the sugar syrup cooks, sift the cornstarch with the cream of tartar. Then stir in the remaining water and mix until dissolved. Pour the mixture into a different saucepan and bring to a boil.
4. When the cornstarch mixture begins to thicken, pour in the sugar syrup.
5. Continue simmering the mixture over low heat for 45 minutes, stirring often to prevent sticking to the bottom of the pan.
6. Remove from heat and stir in the orange water and pistachio.
7. Pour the mixture into a square pan lined with parchment paper.

8. Dust with a bit of cornstarch and let the delight cool and set.
9. Cut into small squares and coat each square in icing sugar.
10. Store the Turkish delight in an airtight container.

Flour Halva Bars

These bars look so pretty, but they are more than just looks. They have the taste, and they are cheap and easy to make!

Time: 2 hours
Servings: 10

Ingredients:

¾ cup coconut oil
2 cups all-purpose flour
2/3 cup white sugar
1 cup cold almond milk
Almonds for topping

Directions:

1. Heat the oil in a heavy saucepan.
2. Stir in the flour and cook for 30 minutes on low heat, stirring often.
3. Gradually stir in the sugar and milk and cook 10 additional minutes.
4. Remove the halva from heat and spoon it into a square pan lined with parchment paper.
5. Level the top as good as possible and let it cool down. Set for a few hours.
6. Cut the halva into small bars and decorate with a few almonds.

Pumpkin Phyllo Rolls

Similar to strudel in terms of how they are made, these rolls are filled with pumpkin and then are flooded in sugar syrup flavored with ginger. What you get is a fragrant and delicious dessert, despite its simplicity!

Time: 1 hour
Servings: 6-8

Ingredients:

1 package phyllo dough sheets
2 pounds pumpkin, peeled and grated
1 teaspoon cinnamon powder
1½ cups water
1½ cups white sugar
1 cinnamon stick
1 teaspoon grated ginger

Directions:

1. Take 2 sheets of phyllo dough and lay them flat on your working surface. Spread a few spoonfuls of grated pumpkin on the dough sheets and roll them tightly.
2. Transfer the roll in a baking tray and repeat with 2 more phyllo dough sheets. Keep going until you run out of dough and pumpkin.
3. Bake in the preheated oven at 350°F for 40 minutes.
4. For the syrup, combine the ingredients in a saucepan and bring to a boil. Cook the syrup until the sugar dissolves then let it cool.
5. When the rolls are done, pour the cold syrup over them and let them soak.
6. Cut into small pieces and serve the rolls chilled.

Carrot Halwa

Carrots have been used for making desserts for decades due to their natural sweetness and amazing flavor. This halwa is one of those rich, fragrant desserts that do them justice!

Time: 1 hour
Servings: 4-6

Ingredients:

 3 cups grated carrot
 2 cups almond milk
 2/3 cup brown sugar
 ¼ cup almond paste
 ½ cup almonds, chopped
 ¼ cup raisins
 2 tablespoons coconut oil

Directions:

1. Combine the carrot and almond milk in a heavy saucepan.
2. Cook on medium flame for 20 minutes then stir in the sugar and coconut oil.
3. Keep cooking until most of the liquid has evaporated.
4. Stir in the almond paste, chopped almonds and raisins then spoon the mixture into individual serving bowls and let it cool completely before serving.

Baklava with Espresso Syrup

Walnuts and coffee are a match made in heaven. No doubt about that! This baklava is a dessert that you'll be making again and again once you take a bite. It's sweet and rich, sticky and fragrant!

Time: 1 hour
Servings: 10

Ingredients:

1 package phyllo dough sheets
½ cup coconut oil
1 pound walnuts, ground
1 cup almond slices
1 teaspoon cinnamon powder
1 teaspoon ground cardamom
1 cup strong brewed coffee
1 cup water
1½ cups sugar

Directions:

1. Mix the walnuts, almond slices, cinnamon and cardamom in a bowl.
2. Layer the phyllo dough sheets with the walnut mixture in a square pan, brushing the dough with coconut oil.
3. Finish with a layer of phyllo dough then cut the baklava into small squares and drizzle it with the remaining coconut oil.
4. Bake in the preheated oven at 350°F for 35-40 minutes or until the top is golden brown.
5. For the syrup, mix coffee, water and sugar in a saucepan. Cook the syrup for 5 minutes.
6. Let the syrup cool down completely.
7. When the baklava is done, remove it from the oven and pour the syrup over it.
8. Let it soak until chilled and serve it fresh.
9. Store it in the fridge.

Pistachio Baklava with Orange Blossom Syrup

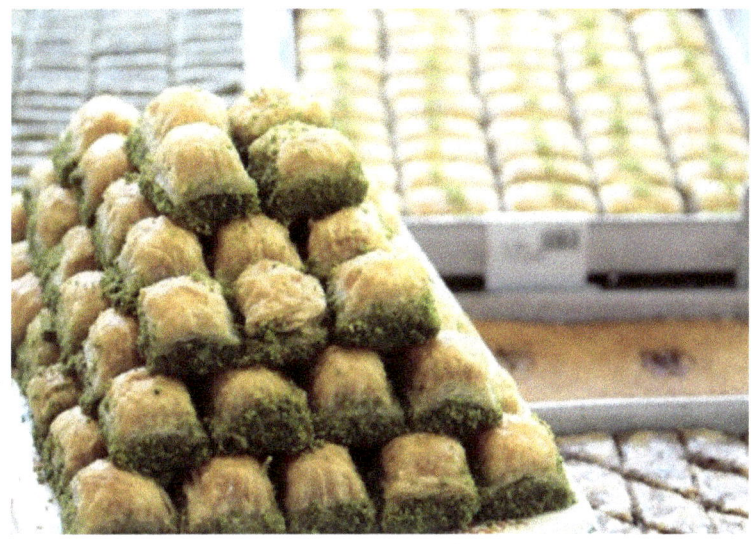

Baklava is generally a very sweet dessert, so you can only eat a bit at a time. But this orange blossom syrup with fresh orange juice balances the sweetness perfectly.

Time: 1 hour
Servings: 10

Ingredients:

- 1 package phyllo dough sheets
- 3 cups ground pistachio
- 1 teaspoon ground cardamom
- 1 tablespoon lemon zest
- ½ cup coconut oil
- 2 cups sugar
- 1 cup water
- ½ cup fresh orange juice
- 1 cinnamon stick
- 1 teaspoon orange blossom water

Directions:

1. To make the syrup, combine the sugar, water, orange juice and cinnamon stick in a saucepan. Cook the syrup for 5 minutes then remove from heat and stir in the orange blossom water. Let the syrup cool completely.
2. Mix the pistachio with cardamom and lemon zest in a bowl.
3. Layer the phyllo sheets and ground pistachio in a square pan. Whilst layering, brush the dough sheets with coconut oil.
4. Finish with a layer of phyllo dough then cut into small squares.
5. Bake in the preheated oven at 350°F for 40 minutes or until golden brown.
6. Remove the baklava from the oven and pour the syrup into the pan.
7. Let the baklava soak up until chilled.
8. Serve the baklava chilled.

Tahini Walnut Cookies

Crisp and crumbly, these cookies are the perfect treat to serve with a cup of Turkish coffee!

Time: 1 hour
Servings: 4 dozen

Ingredients:

¼ cup sesame oil
½ cup tahini paste
1 cup vegetable oil
1 cup sugar
1 teaspoon vanilla extract
1 cup ground walnuts
3 cups all-purpose flour
1 pinch salt

Directions:

1. Combine all the ingredients in a food processor. Pulse until well mixed and an easy-to-work-with dough is formed.
2. Form small balls and place them on baking trays lined with parchment paper.
3. Flatten the balls with a fork and bake in the preheated oven at 350°F for 15-20 minutes or until golden brown and crisp on the edges.
4. Let the cookies cool completely before serving.
5. Store them in an airtight container for up to 2 weeks.

Preserved Figs

This recipe preserves the amazing and delicate flavor of figs, so you can enjoy them even out of season!

Time: 40 minutes
Yields: 1 jar

Directions:

  8 medium size figs
  1 large glass jar
  ½ cup white sugar
  1 cup water
  1 cup fresh orange juice
  2 orange peels
  1 star anise
  2 cardamom pods

Directions:

1. Combine all the ingredients in a glass jar and seal it with a lid.
2. Place the jar in a deep saucepan then pour cold water in the pan until it covers ¾ of the jar.
3. Boil for 30 minutes then turn the heat off and let the figs cool in the water.
4. Store the preserved figs for a few months in a cold place.

Cardamom Poached Figs

Although not as famous as the poached pears, these poached figs are still delicious! They turn slightly tender and infuse with the cardamom aroma. They are best served chilled!

Time: 35 minutes
Servings: 2-4

Ingredients:

1 pounds fresh figs
4 green cardamom pods, crushed
¼ cup brandy
1 vanilla pod, cut in half lengthwise
2 cups water
¼ cup brown sugar

Directions:

1. Combine cardamom, brandy, vanilla, water and sugar in a saucepan and bring to a boil.
2. Add the figs and cook for 15 minutes until tender.
3. Serve the poached pears chilled.

Burnt Bottom Pudding

In its essence, this dessert is a pudding, but what makes it special is the burnt bottom which adds a delicate smoky aroma to the creamy, delicious dessert.

Time: 1 hour
Servings: 10

Ingredients:

6 cups almond milk
¼ cup rice flour
¾ cup cornstarch
1 cup sugar
1 teaspoon vanilla extract
¼ cup sugar

Directions:

1. Mix the flours together in a bowl. Stir in 1 cup of almond milk and mix until well combined and there are no lumps.
2. Bring the remaining milk to a boil in a heavy saucepan. Stir in the sugar.
3. Add the flour mixture and mix until the pudding begins to thicken.
4. Remove from heat and stir in the vanilla.
5. Pour the pudding into the bowl of a stand mixer and keep mixing on low speed until the caramel is ready.
6. For the caramel, melt the sugar in a heavy saucepan. Add the coconut oil.
7. Take 1 cup of pudding and pour it over the caramel. It will sizzle and burn slightly.
8. Remove from heat and let the burnt layer set for 5 minutes then pour the remaining pudding into the pan as well.
9. Let the pudding set for a few hours then turn it upside down on a platter.
10. Serve it chilled.

Rice Flour Pudding

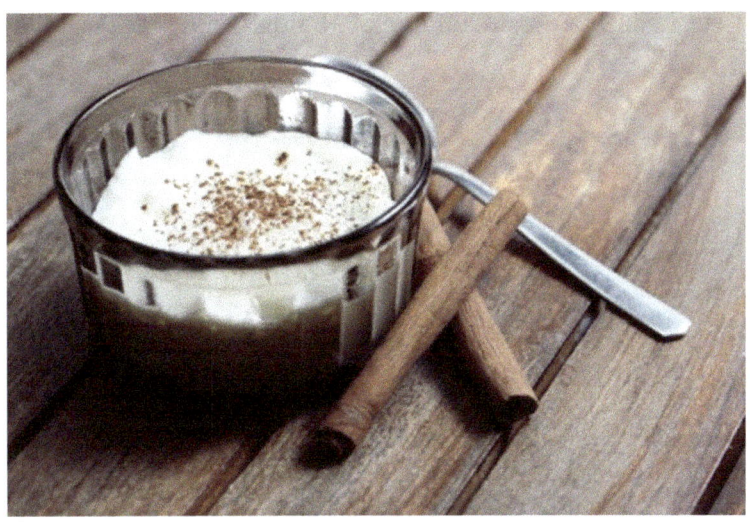

Rice flour is a great thickener for desserts, but it's also nutritious and filling. In addition to that, it cooks easily so if you feel like having a pudding for dessert today, choose this recipe! Top it with chopped nuts and you've got yourself a complete dessert that is creamy and textured at the same time!

Time: 30 minutes
Servings: 2-4

Ingredients:

  2 cups almond milk
  ¼ cup sugar
  3 tablespoons rice flour
  ½ teaspoon orange blossom water

Directions:

1. Mix the milk and sugar in a saucepan.
2. Bring the mixture to a boil over low heat then stir in the rice flour.
3. Mix the pudding well with a whisk until it begins to thicken.

4. Stir in the orange blossom water and pour the pudding into individual serving bowls.
5. Let the pudding cool completely before serving.

Conclusion

The Turkish cuisine appears to be one of the main columns of the world's cuisine. Its use of spices, dried fruits and nuts, as well as innovative ways of cooking vegetables set it apart as a distinguished cuisine. You don't need to be originated from Turkey to enjoy this kind of food, but you do need a taste for spices, grains and vegetables, a taste for unusual soups and fragrant stews, a taste for rich main dishes and innovative appetizers. Turkish cuisine is a complete and nutritious one, and a book like this one can only be a gain in your kitchen!

Lightning Source UK Ltd.
Milton Keynes UK
UKHW021435101220
374890UK00005B/100